Living My Life Like It's Golden

Believe It OR Not, I Made It & You Can Too

Angela Johnson

Publishing Services by Stanton Publishing House

ISBN: 9781712255766(KDP AMAZON)
ISBN: 9781078748988(BARNES & NOBLE)
Library of Congress Control Number: 2019919306

Dedication

I want to dedicate this book to anyone who struggles with disability and mental illness.

Contents

Introduction

I am Angela Johnson. I am thirty-seven years old, and I live in the rural area of Greenwood, Mississippi. I have four children and have been happily married for fourteen years. I will talk more about my children and husband later throughout my book. This book is the story of my life.

My life has been filled with a mixture of hardships and happiness. Sometimes, my life seems to get a little off balance. Who I am and how I was raised are essential factors in the way I now live. Getting the strength to write this book demonstrates my growth as a person and my growth as someone who was born brain-damaged, with a learning and speech disability. Growing up, being brain-damaged on my left side and having hyperthyroidism was challenging, and I became more comfortable and easier to cope with as I grew and found myself.

Chapter 1

Many people have their lucky numbers, but I was characterized as the lucky 'Seven' of my nine siblings, in a large but beautiful family that my loving parents, Jefferey and Violet brought up. Baptist Town was where I was born and raised, specifically brought to this world at the Greenwood Leflore Hospital.

The sibling bond I had with my brothers and sisters wasn't always the best, but somehow, the days in the 'shotgun' house were filled with fun and joy; the house was something I would never forget and the long-lasting memories I had there.

My siblings and I didn't grow up close, but we had a sibling bond no matter the circumstances – always being there for one another.

I could vividly remember one of the many bad memories of my childhood: them and other kids calling me out of my name.

They always made fun of me because of my disabilities, and because I had constant seizures. The words used, "You aren't gon' be shit," "Retard," and "Ha-ha, you can't talk," hurt badly, and they left deep scars in my soul. How can someone have such an amount of hatred within them, especially from my blood siblings?

Crying was normal to me, to the point where I fell asleep with tears in my eyes. At the same time, I asked God, "Why me?" Seeking the fault in myself, until I grew to realize that how others treated me was not my fault.

Ultimately, I ended up distancing myself to avoid the mistreatment. My mother, on the other hand, wanted me to get surgery. I could still remember her telling me how the doctors would cut my brain open to performing a dangerous operation. My grandmother was opposed to that and said, "I believe in her; if it's the Lord's will, then she'll be just fine with prayer."

I knew I would be different from other children for the rest of my life, but I was comforted with the fact that everything would be okay, life was something beautiful to look forward to, and I was starting to shape mine. My grandmother was a wise lady. She was known for her thoughtful advice, so she always advised my mother to keep her faith because things weren't always as they looked like, and there was a lot that neither of them understood.

Getting the surgery wasn't my destiny, and as the years had passed, things began to look a little better.

Like every child, I was more than attached to my mother growing up, always being by her side. My sister, Mia, took care of me before I could walk and helped bathe me; she helped out in the most important things that brought warmth to my heart. While other kids disregarded me, she would play with me. At the age of five, I started to talk, and then later on, when I turned eight, I was able to walk.

People always criticized me, like I was some mistake. I've always felt different, and at that time, I didn't know that being different was something beautiful. When I started school, my classmates always voiced their opinions, which were the ultimate worst.

Skylar, my sister, came to my defense and always tried to fight them; while my sister, Mia, also couldn't hold back and told everyone that I was sick, stating how they didn't have a right to talk wrong about me.

I always had a strong faith in God; I always had questions such as, "Why me?" I was filled with anger, but I was also born in a world of sin; anyway, nobody was perfect on this earth. The best answer to my question would be that God gave the most challenging battles to his best soldiers.

He helped me the most; my faith didn't bring me down a second or disappoint me. People didn't know me or what I was suffering, yet they judged me. My mother was a single mother but always provided us with everything we needed.

As time passed and I got much better, we moved from Baptist Town to Rising Sun, then to Leflore Avenue. However, the most beautiful home was on Leflore Avenue, where we had a big white house, and it was much more modern than the others.

After we moved to that house, we got the tragic news of my father passing away; the cause of death was poison; at least that was what I was told.

Life for me started when I was fifteen; that's when I first got in the streets and experienced what many kids my age did, sneaking out of the house, skipping school, and doing many other things I wasn't allowed to do. It was relatively early for a fifteen-year-old to do those things, but I just wanted to live my life with freedom.

I didn't have much guidance to know right from wrong because my mother was an alcoholic, and it wasn't the best environment. Being at home was miserable. I had the urge to run away but knew it wasn't the best idea.

The alcohol got to my mother and soon became a big problem; she sold the house and moved to Memphis, Tennessee, while she left us with Mia. I maintained the house, being the most responsible and reasonable one.

Being so attached to my mother early on led to me being hurt when she left, but I was even more hurt when she didn't attend my high school graduation. I was left speechless, confused as to why she would do that. I was her daughter.

While everyone's family attended their graduation, she wasn't there, present. A little after that had happened, she moved back to our house. I couldn't be mad at her for long even though her actions so angered me; I took the good with the bad.

Receiving bad news was something regular; while I was on my yearly check-up, my doctor told me that because of my health condition, I wouldn't be able to have children; that was the moment the world ended for me. Children are what most people look forward to, starting their own families, watching them grow but for me, that wouldn't be the case. I was devastated and crying beyond measure.

I was grateful my family was there to comfort me; they tried to make me feel better by saying if that were God's plan, I would have kids. Then not much to my knowledge, a miracle had worked in my life when I least expected it. I went to the doctor when I felt sick the next month and when the results came, it turned out that I was two weeks pregnant.

I couldn't believe it! Shock took over me as I kept asking the doctor if he was sure. Yes, I was pregnant, and it was one of the best moments I had ever experienced. I wasn't ready to tell my mother yet and tried my best to hide it from her. I wasn't sure how she would react; would she be mad or happy for me? But when I finally had some courage and decided to tell her, she told me that she already knew.

She said that she could tell when one of her girls was pregnant. She told me that she was happy for me because being pregnant was the best gift God could give me. She also told me that she was very displeased when she found out how my baby's father reacted.

My baby's father claimed that I was lying and screamed at me that it wasn't his baby, claiming he was done with me. On January 09, I gave birth to my son, Billy, an 8.25-pound baby boy. My family was there by my side, and it was a blessing. I was beyond grateful for my family.

Billy father asked for a blood test, and the results came back positive – 99.99% of his child. I didn't want him in my son's life; I was enraged by how he treated me during the pregnancy and decided not to have anything to do with him anymore. I had enough brothers, and they all stepped in and became father figures for my son.

I kept hoping I would someday find my soul mate, this life wasn't meant for only suffering, and while I was taking care of my son, I couldn't help but feel lonely at the same time. Suddenly, a guy named Oliver came into my life. The five-year age gap wasn't much, but our chemistry was something else; we were meant for each other.

It brought me comfort how he never questioned me, my child, or my decisions; it was something fresh I had never experienced before. However, our families were opposed to our relationship, claiming a five-year age difference was too much.

The complex we later moved into wasn't much, and we called it the "Coca-Cola" plant. We didn't need anything high end, we only needed one another, and it was more than enough; we soon moved to Snowden Jones Apartments.

The years we spent together were magical; we knew we were meant for each other, and eventually, we decided to get married; Oliver being only eighteen, while I was twenty-three. As I previously said, age didn't matter to us since the love we felt was much more substantial. On June 05, 2004, my husband and I exchanged vows; I was sure that was the best day of my life; we had made it through it all, the doubts and the negativity from the outside. I felt complete; we had made it.

Our bond was strong, nobody could break it, and we learned to stick together through everything. Oliver truly cared about me. I could feel it and see it by his actions, more than anyone else in my life.

Oliver accepted my son as his own, which I was grateful for, and my son also liked him too, which made me extremely happy. My life had a purpose, and it was just starting to shape into something beautiful.

It was the best decision to enroll Billy in day-care. One day, while he was attending, we received a horrifying call that had me at a total loss for words, shocked, while a million thoughts rushed through my head, not very optimistic. I was informed that he had not woken up from his nap; he wasn't necessarily tired, which worried me the most; I was on high alert and panicking.

They said they had called the ambulance and had to take him to the hospital because he was experiencing abnormal heartbeats.

I showed up at the clinic to discover my child being determined to have paroxysmal supraventricular tachycardia (PSVT).

Ordinarily, an electrical sign is produced in uncommon pacemaker cells in the upper office of the heart. This motivation makes the chamber beat in an organized manner and drives blood into the ventricles.

The electrical signal continues to a junction box between the atrium and ventricle, where there is a slight delay. It permits the chamber to contract and send blood to the ventricle. The sign proceeds all through the ventricles and makes them beat and push blood to the body. In paroxysmal supraventricular tachycardia, irregular conduction of that power causes the chamber, and optionally the ventricles, to beat quickly.

It is paroxysmal because the quick rate can happen irregularly and abruptly. After that episode, I viewed my child intently and dropped by his day-care from time to time to keep an eye on him. He required medicine each day due to his condition. I watched him to an ever-increasing extent. I used to be frightened for him to play with many kids, "harsh" kids, to be specific. I began to feel a lot more cautious about whom he was playing with when he was outside.

Eventually, we moved to Athens, Georgia, which is known for its antebellum architecture. I wanted a change with so much going on; I was tired of living the same monotone life and needed to encounter new things and carry on with a somewhat unique way of life.

Life in Athens was so much better; we moved and discovered our way around quickly. Oliver got a decent paying position, and I did as well. Things were going incredibly well. My child was growing, and obviously, my family was as well.

Later, I found out that I was pregnant with my second child; it was a girl, and I was beyond excited. Being pregnant again eased both me and my work exertion down. I wanted to enjoy my pregnancy, and the growing belly caused me to slow down with work and be a stay at home mom, while my husband worked most days and some nights.

It was difficult. I was grateful for my husband working so much, but I could barely take care of my child and I seeing as I was pregnant. Besides everything, I enjoyed life in Athens; it brought me peace.

Life was alright up until one dreadful day in early October when my brother, Jason, my older brother, Billy, Oliver and my son Billy, headed to the local Wal-Mart. It was a day I would never forget, a tragedy.

I made the harrowing mistake of leaving my phone on the roof of the car; while we were riding, it slid on the windshield in front of us, and I couldn't help but yell out, "Damn it, my phone!" My childish mistake made us pull over to get it. Jason, my brother, insisted on getting it even though Oliver came out with him.

I watched as Jason got out onto the freeway, my world stopped, and my heart dropped at the sudden sight of him being hit by a car. The driver that hit him had barely noticed; I watched as they dragged my baby brother down the freeway, a painful sight that would haunt me.

Another driver pulled over to help us and called an ambulance immediately. I was shaking, and in shock, my heart was beating out of its average pace, as I tried to take in what had just happened.

I immediately thought my brother was dead, and it was my entire fault. I was crying uncontrollably, while Skylar was so angry that she viciously cursed at me. The sight in front of me terrorized me; I watched them pick up his flesh off the ground in horror. They loaded him on a stretcher with no tongue, and a hanging ear, and nose, drenched in blood. God was by his side that day and spared him.

It was a miracle that he was stable; however, I wasn't. That day would haunt me, and I had reoccurring dreams of the accident. The stress and worry I went through daily, weren't any good for me, and I was going on eight months of being pregnant.

Before I knew it, I was rushed to the Athens Regional Hospital. I would have my baby with my family by my side, supporting me. There wasn't stopping my baby girl, who decided to come early, but as soon as I pushed her out that day, she had stopped breathing; the nurses took her to ICU, and it was more than my heart could take.

I was tired of it. I prayed to God to bless my child; I only wanted her to be healthy. She was born weighing two pounds. I called her my little soldier, so little but so brave. She was named Niyah Nicole by my niece, Kaylee.

I was released to go home, but I wasn't going with my daughter; she had to stay there for another month, which I understood. Besides everything, I was at the hospital most of the time. I spent time with her and my husband.

I could vividly remember having to put on gloves to hold her while she was in the incubator, I was overjoyed seeing her doing better, and it brought a smile to my face. She was deprived of oxygen during birth, and currently, she has asthma and a speech problem. I loved her beyond words.

We finally got the chance to take home our little soldier at the end of the month. Oliver has had to work harder to support the kids and me, while I was taking care of the children alone at home. We found ourselves moving back to Mississippi, where my mother could help me look after the kids. We moved to Greenwood's Jordan Lane and bought our first home.

I had many thoughts and lots of things going on; things eventually got worse when we started being unfaithful towards each other. I was the first to make a mistake and didn't know what exactly happened in our relationship to lead me to that.

It was a guy from Walthall Street that I cheated on him with; by the time Oliver had found out, his pride was hurt, and he was angry, wanting to fight the guy because he was feeling so mad. Somehow, I managed to convince him that I would leave the guy alone and not talk to him again.

I was happy in my marriage, but he needed to make me feel what I did when I first met him; he must've thought that money made me happy because he was working all the time and always made sure I had his pay checks.

Oliver was my husband; I hoped it wasn't too late to realize my mistake and how he didn't deserve to be treated like that. "Selfish" was the word to describe me the best at that time.

He gave me a second chance, and we made up, which led to us making up more than we intended to because I found myself pregnant again. I prayed for a healthy baby, my thoughts being in the scares I had experienced with my previous two kids.

I gave birth to a healthy baby girl on January 24, 2009, naming her Na'Kayla Shanice. My world was complete with having them all at home. I now had my three children, and my husband.

Unfortunately, my happiness didn't last as long as I wanted it to. It was time for my husband to pay back the heartbreak I caused him, and he left me. I was left alone with my children, while he moved in with another woman, leaving me shattered.

I had lost my will to function, I couldn't eat or sleep. My mind was always on him; I was heartbroken. One day, he abruptly called, asking about the kids. I told him the truth that they were missing their dad and called him out on leaving me. I told him how hard it was for me to take care of my kids with my condition, and after that conversation, he moved back with us.

I felt complete and forgave him entirely for leaving me; things were going back to normal, as they were supposed to.

I couldn't forget what he did to me. His infidelity was always on my mind, and it kept lingering around as much as I wanted it to pass. While we worked things out, we moved into an even bigger house.

Our family was back on track, functioning correctly as a healthy family should. What bothered me was when I noticed that he was starting to go out more and was hanging out with his friend, which was strange. Our relationship was based on trust, and I didn't want to have any second thoughts, but I didn't know how to feel and began to worry. Something felt off, even though I fully trusted him.

I could recollect a specific day as if it happened yesterday. My husband was spending time with his cousin, Eric, and as he came back home, he sat in the yard to relax. He claimed they had just left from walking around the fair and saw Kaylee there, my niece. I didn't give it much importance and went on with my day, walking back in the house and surfing the web.

A sudden abrupt noise from outside my house caught my attention, and I instantly got up to my feet to check who it was. To my shock, I came face to face with the "other" woman. I was fuming with anger but didn't show a sign of it; I was calm and recollected in front of her, only asking what she wanted. I instantly assumed it was because of Oliver.

She was visibly bothered by me and looked like she was about to fight me. She informed me that they had been messing around for six months while we were separated. Then, she rolled up her shirt to show me the name tattooed on her. My husband's name was permanently inked on her body; it angered me beyond measure. How did she have the right to do this? I could not believe her.

I was ready, and it was on; my rage was through the roof, and I didn't hold back. She couldn't even utter a word before I charged at her. I had an adrenaline rush, which didn't let me stop anytime soon, a blow-for-blow. I was determined to let my anger out, and I noticed Oliver's sister had joined my side, jumping in and helping me fight her; fighting and grappling her was something to be seen.

My family was shocked by my actions but knew there was a reason behind it; she had pissed me off. I never usually fought, but this was something else. Oliver was scared and hidden away in the doghouse; he was afraid I would divorce him, leave and take my children with me, but that wasn't the case. He begged me to stay with him, reassuring me he was sorry and didn't want to ruin what we had in our marriage.

I wanted to put everything behind us, and that's what I told him. His father had stopped by our house after everything had gone down and advised us to work on our love, fight for our marriage. Love was more potent than anything, and if we did love each other, we wouldn't give up to save what's worth saving.

Mistakes were meant to be made; we had to be open with discussing our problems regularly, not holding back. My father-in-law told us that everybody made mistakes and everybody had flaws, but it was up to us to give people a chance and start over again.

It was a wake-up call for Oliver and me since we listened to him very well. We started putting ourselves first, focusing on what was going on in our family rather than outside in the streets; spending more time together was necessary. We did; taking trips and visiting places we always wanted to go to, even going to Las Vegas.

It was a healthy shift for us, and I wanted it to continue. Vegas was magical and what had happened there had to be said to our family; I realized my love for him was much more significant than I thought; we did have our ups and downs but so did many couples. We remained together through it all and have three beautiful kids who we love to the moon and back.

Life was giving us its blessings, and after all, there was a bright path in front of us.

Chapter 2

The relationship my parents had wasn't the best. They were always on and off and leading different lives. One time, they were together, and the next day, separated. My father had a separate life when I was twelve and had a completely different family, already married to another woman.

He didn't miss out on our lives and stopped by to check on me and my siblings, still caring about how and what we were doing. His wife, who I got a chance to meet, was graceful, very nice, and respectful, so I called her "Momma," and wasn't alone, and my siblings did too.

My mother was the epitome of a strong independent woman, who I looked up to and adored. She didn't need a man in her life to validate her and be the reason for her happiness; she brought us up well on her own, which was impressive.

Jason and Demario were her favorites, her boys, and nobody could've said anything wrong about them; she would always defend them no matter what. Each one of us had a distinctive personality, specifically the girls. Mia was destined to be successful, either acting appropriately or studying; she was the best in almost everything she did, and I admired her.

On the other hand, when I needed help with something, she was the one I always called, or Skylar, getting on their nerves daily. Skylar was much more different than Mia, always getting into fights and arguing with someone around the corner; my mom still liked the girls, but sometimes, we seemed to have a lot more going on than the boys, and she didn't know how to handle it. Billy and everyone else, with their own stories and prerogatives, had my mother's hands full.

With my mom and dad being separated, she was single up until she met this man named Jason. He was my younger brother's father, and he was named after him, Jason Author. I thought he was the right choice for my mother; they complemented one another entirely, just as they were two peas in a pod, twin souls if you asked me.

I wouldn't say they were raging alcoholics, but they liked their "liquor;" they were together all of the time, and they frequently went to the club in Baptist Town. You could see Jason in my mother in just a glance; I wondered how it was possible to love someone that much, but I saw it in my mother's eyes and the news that she was about to deliver another offspring, the root of their love was born on July of 1990, the baby boy was named Jason Author, Jr, but we called him "Blue." He was and always will be the brightest one in our family; he had sandy brown hair and hazel eyes, slightly tall. Everyone else in our family was either dark or a medium caramel looking color.

Blue was a somewhat troublesome kid growing up, all of those whippings toughened him up, which caused him to mature early on, and all of us had our own thing going on. There was Marshall, who was barely at home; Mia, who fought to make something out of herself and succeed in life; Billy was the madman, the craziest one of us all, while Carlo's main focus was making money. Skylar was trouble, the tomboy and a streetfighter; then there was me, the one who they all made fun of. Even after it all, I felt that I deserved a chance and made something out of myself; I wanted them to respect me. My mother sure put up with a lot with raising us at the time.

My mom's relationship with Jason didn't last, and they soon separated with him moving to Memphis, Tennessee, with his family, while my mother did her best to raise us in Mississippi.

I could remember the day before Blue's birthday vividly; a storm had passed over Memphis, knocking the power out. His dad, Jason Author, had a severe asthma attack, and due to him not being able to get his medicine, he passed away.

We didn't know how to break the news to Blue, it was on his birthday, and we had to tell him the worst news ever. The news changed him entirely, and it was a tragedy, which he couldn't get over; my mother had the strength to continue raising us on her own.

Chapter 3

I always wondered how my brother, Jamari, was so good at so many things, especially at basketball. I would describe him as big and tall; you would instantly notice him in a crowded room. He just stood out, a fighter and a lover; a rather impressive combination for such a kid.

Being so independent at such a young age, he moved in with our grandmother, Leola; there was something special about him and the way he carried himself. He did leave us, but at the same time, I thought it was a good thing.

He had the opportunity to become a professional basketball player. I thought it was because he was older and how he was getting treated; either way, I wished the best for my brother.

Today, Jamari has four children, and all of them are boys. He is leading a happy married life with his wife, Faith, and they have been together for many years now.

Marshall was one of us who were slightly reserved. He liked to keep to himself the most, but that didn't mean he didn't like to have fun. Twelve years of his life, he spent in jail, and it seemed that his nerves had expired there; he had a bad temper.

He was something else, different from each one of us. He settled down in Athens, Georgia, and got married, with step-children.

My brother, Demario, was also incarcerated during his lifetime and spent twelve years of his life in jail. He was in prison during his son's birthday named after him, Demario Jr. His son and his wife were spending their days alone, without him.

Due to him being unable to see his family and not spending any time with them, he and his wife had filed for a divorce. The man didn't wait long until he remarried another woman. As time passed, he was released from prison and only sentenced to five years on paper. Once he was released, his attitude towards us was changed. I was not too fond of it one bit, as if we owed him something. I wouldn't say I liked it at all.

In my teenage years, my sister, Skylar, was mainly influenced; even though I was the older one, she made me do many things and break out of my shell. She was loyal, something else. Even when I got my first tattoo, she was right there by my side. By the time I was introduced to the streets, so was she.

Even though we were different, I felt like she was another version of me, a mini-me but with a better functioning mind.

With almost all of my siblings bullying me as I was growing up, I could barely get along with any of them, but with her, it was somehow different. I trusted her the most, and she knew most of my secrets. We always had each other's backs no matter what; we were partners in crime, and I was grateful she made my teenage years wild. We snuck out of the house together and even took beatings for one another; it was a ride or die situation for us. We had that special bond that was unbreakable. However, Mia was much different and rarely hung out with us. She didn't want to get in trouble and focused on herself.

Running the streets so young affected her when she was fifteen and she found out she was pregnant. Right before her birthday, she gave birth to one of the cutest and handsome little boy. She named him Keller.

Skylar's kidneys failed on her when she had the baby, and it came to everyone's shock that they were coding my sister, still grateful to God she was able to survive. Having a son didn't stop her from returning to her old life; she didn't slow down one bit and continued where she left off. I don't blame her, although I did blame my mother.

My mother was the one who took care of him the most, as if he was her son and not Skylar's. Later on, my sister found love and got married. What came as news after that was her being pregnant again, and this time around, it was a girl. She gave birth to the most beautiful girl I had ever seen and named her Brooklyn, after her father.

Skylar's life drastically changed when she and her husband moved to Athens, Georgia. The rest of our family was still in Greenwood, and I could still recall the harrowing day we got the call that Skylar was shot in the head by her husband.

Almost everyone who lived in Greenwood came to the house that I had on Jordan Street and tried to comfort me in the best way possible. I was crying uncontrollably and kept asking God why he let that happen.

Most of all, we all kept asking ourselves how her husband could be so ruthless and such an evil person to do such a thing. We soon got the information that the story was mixed up due to our long-distance; my sister was shot in the leg and not her head. Even though it wasn't as fatal, it was still something that my family couldn't get over. Someone whom we all thought loved her, shot her to death, or so we thought.

Our family was still heated and angry, ready to go on an old-fashioned search, but he was lucky he was arrested, and my sister came back to Greenwood. It was all jokes when she came back, claiming her being so harsh and finally getting a war-wound; besides everything, I was glad my sister was safe and could move on from the traumatic experience.

Today, Skylar is still living in Greenwood, MS., and her husband is still incarcerated.

The one who was considered the most successful in my family was my sister, Mia. Due to her being so independent and well-spoken, many people tend to mistake her for a lawyer when she is a social worker and has been for some time now.

She was somewhat different in the right way. She had her days when she would come by and hang out with everyone, and some days, she would just rather chill at home and sit by herself. Mia was blessed with three children, Kaylee, Kelly, and Savannah. Kaylee is twenty-seven, Kelly is twenty-five, and Savannah is sixteen. They are all beautiful young people, and she loves them to death.

My sister spoils Savannah the most, being the baby. I wouldn't say Kaylee and Kelly got the same treatment, but she had a soft spot for her youngest daughter. Kaylee moved out when she was seventeen and moved in with Skylar; when she turned nineteen, she moved into her boyfriend's place.

Kelly took a different path in life, and as soon as he turned seventeen, he joined the military, being currently at his Basic Combat training in South Carolina. Mia was going through a life crisis.

My brother, Carlo, who goes by the name of Lil Digger, loved his money and would do anything to get it; I would judge him as a slick and cheerful person, always being realistic with everyone, which is a good trait.

He always comes up with the most reasonable, mature thoughts and likes being idealistic, while he talks sense into someone. Sometimes, he would annoy our family members by pushing buttons that] don't want to be pushed, but with that being his nature, nobody got mad at him for long.

The brother I could relate to the most out of my siblings was Billy; he was older than Carlo but younger than Demario. While growing up, he also had a speech problem; he stuttered severely but was still fun to be around and always had the best stories to tell us.

Billy didn't have any limits when working; he went to work and got drunk when he wanted to. He was a positive person who was always cool with everyone. I named my son after him. Everyone shared my opinion about him being a calm person; they loved him.

Chapter 4

Coping with a mental disability wasn't easy. I felt like I was all alone most of the time. However, things weren't always like that; your surroundings and family depend on it to get much more potent and to understand that it doesn't define you. If you have a supportive family, feel blessed.

If that's not the case for you and you don't have a supportive family, your journey may be a lot harder than the rest. This book is made for me to help you cope with your situation, reflect on your life, and establish a mind-frame to not care about what anyone else says.

Others say it doesn't define you, so when somebody calls you ugly, you tell yourself that you're beautiful. Beauty is in the eye of the beholder; how you feel about yourself is far more important than how someone else feels about you.

You have to put yourself first, and even though you don't feel loved by someone, you should still love yourself; before loving someone else, you have to love yourself.

This world is what you make of it; at first it may seem that everything is messed up, but you have to sit by yourself and think about the nice things and your future, where you want to be and see yourself in that better place. Surely it will bring your mood up, and things will turn to positive.

Those who talk about others don't like themselves; even if they say some emotionless words to you, they shouldn't hurt because they do not come from someone worthy of you. Those who think you need help are usually those needing help themselves.

You will have to go against mean and prejudiced people your whole life; unfortunately, that's how the world works. Some people can't help but be mean and rude; it reflects how they were raised and how they were treated throughout their life.

I was raised brain-damaged, with many family issues and problems; however, I later shaped myself as a person, but not once did I offend or judge anyone.

You have to create a mind-frame where you believe in yourself when no one else wants to.

Creating your reality and being positive is one of the most critical keys in shaping yourself.

Do not give up on yourself; the number one rule to succeed. When you find yourself going through some problems, if you don't have anyone to talk to or be there for you, be there for yourself and try to surround yourself with positive people. Always prioritise quality over quantity.

You don't want any negative people in your life; they have no business in telling you what's right and what's wrong. Those types of people give advice that's for the best in their interest, not for you. Once you separate yourself, you are going to see a real change.

It's hard when due to the lack of communication skills, your family and other people decide to ignore you. You feel alone as if nobody in the world can understand what you're going through. Being pessimistic about your situation isn't an option; you have to learn to rise above it and go against people who don't believe in you. If you feel alone, ask God to advise and lead your path into a positive mindset.

"Why me?" Was the question I often asked myself when in reality, I should've been asking, "Why not me?" Even though I had to go through so much, I was destined to go through it. I was made in the image of my creator. I am slowly finding my purpose on this earth and learning that God doesn't make any mistakes.

Being different than everyone else doesn't make you worthless; you are still human, and there is nothing wrong with you. There may be some instances where you feel out of place and lack self-esteem, but at the end of the day, you're unique and special.

Most of the time, you will find yourself wanting to be alone, you won't know how to express your feelings to the fullest, which is one of the reasons you keep most of your problems to yourself, but you have to find someone to trust and tell how you feel. Everyone does deserve time to themselves, but in your case, keeping so many things bottled up could be fatal mentally.

Don't hold back. Say what's on your mind; find a friend who is worth it and who listens to you. It will change your life.

Take therapy if you need to, don't be afraid to take action to better your own life. I go to Life Help Mental Health Center for therapy for my depression and anger at my family for maltreating me, and also for all the bullying that I experienced in high school.

Life Help Mental Health taught me many things, and helped me through so much. I wouldn't be here without their help. I was diagnosed with bipolar disorder and depression.

Chapter 5

I n life, you will need someone to be there for you during hard times, someone who is going to be your shoulder to cry on, protect you and provide for you. Here, your quest for love begins; I've been told many times that I should let love find me, but it made me think that they didn't want me to find anyone. Many people will not want a person with a disability.

That's the problem in modern society; we are obsessed with looks and we forget what's inside, what matters. We are looking for someone perfect when, in reality, that someone doesn't exist; nobody is perfect.

I wasn't looking for love when I met my husband, but somehow, I found my soul mate. It all happened so suddenly that it didn't surprise me. I went through some awful things that I felt I deserved when I found the love. He was the man who could love, provide, and protect me. He was everything I wanted.

Once you find the one, you need to make sure they will be there for you through thick and thin. Find out whether they are willing to give up their life to become a member of yours. Although not many, those are the main qualities that I looked for: loyal, faithful, honest, respect.

As I said earlier, you should love yourself even if no one else does; here, you have to apply the same thing, always putting yourself first and believing in yourself so that if things don't work out at the end of the day, you would still feel fulfilled.

This life will be filled with people who take you for granted and people who take advantage of you, but there will be a time when they realize what they had; you never know what you had until it's gone.

For me, giving up was an option; many times, I found myself tired and on the verge of doing so, but I didn't, neither should you. Giving up is not worth it. Keep on pushing for a better life, stick it out and do the best you can with the life that you already have.

Relationships sometimes become complicated; there're conflicts, fights, jealousy, and it may seem like you don't understand each other at all. You may have second thoughts about your relationship, not knowing where it may lead. Sometimes, it may be right for you, but sometimes, not. You have to find someone who will understand your situation; someone who will love you and are there for you forever.

Unfortunately, some people like to take advantage of us. They mean us no good in a relationship. You know the ones I'm talking about: those who stick around to spend your disability checks at the first of the month, pretending to love you. Those are the people to be the most careful of. They are dirty enough to try to trick you into believing that they love you, yet they want to get your money.

Money shouldn't be a priority for the person who loves you; they need to love you for you, no matter your past or current condition. Someone who will only look forward to the future and forget the past.

Reading my words, you may think that finding real love is hard, but it's not in reality. It sneaks up on you when you least expect it, and it's called, 'fate.' However, you shouldn't take anyone's love for granted. You shouldn't be hung up on your past relationships, thinking your new one won't work; everyone is not alike; everyone is different, and you should view them as such. The past is called the past for a reason.

Chapter 6

Finding the right person for you may take a while; in the meantime, try to take care and focus more on yourself. Make yourself happy first before trying to make someone else. You must treat yourself, and do things you wouldn't normally do. Making yourself feel loved is very important.

Trust and love always go together; you can't love someone without trusting them. Those words always go together. If you have second thoughts about trusting someone while you love them, I don't feel like you genuinely love that person.

When you love someone, you must love them as you love yourself. Loving yourself comes first, always. If you're not able to love yourself, you won't be able to love someone else.

Marriage is ruled out to be the goal in a relationship; that's how society works. If you're in love, you get married, but those values vanished in modern society. Many people find themselves having a lot of trust issues in marriage and relationships. Those who are married are far from happy, seeking happiness outside of their marriage.

Precisely what happened to me. While having special needs, you need to be extra cautious about these things and seek someone who will love you and not what you have. Exchanging vows is essential; you're asked to love each other through sickness and health, for richer and poorer, till death does you apart. However, today that's not the case, and those vows are being taken for granted, like "Good-morning," "Hello," and "How-do-you-do" messages. Many leave their significant others in sickness, resulting in financial instability.

Being disabled doesn't mean you are "lesser" in life; that should be the reason for striving to be more significant, looking forward to what God has in store for you. Marriages are sacred and should never be based on sex, money, and material things. They should be based on bringing out the best in each other, trust, faithfulness, and most important of all, love.

The one who loves you shouldn't bring you down, judge you or mistreat you; if they do, it only shows that they are not meant for you and that they are bringing out your worst.

As the Serenity Prayers state: you must accept the things that you cannot change, change the things that you can, and have the wisdom to know the difference. If you're not treated right, get out of the relationship. This world has way too many people for you to be hung up on one, even though you're utterly in love with them, scars heal, but they can't heal if you won't let them.

You have to be smart and not let these people manipulate you; once you find 'the one,' you will know by what you feel.

Please don't give up entirely on someone. Try to give them time; maybe they are worth saving. No one is perfect, and you should not go around looking for someone who is. If you are looking for the perfect person, you'll be looking forever.

You can go ahead and get used to people coming in and out of your life and you being disappointed. There are imperfect people who will be perfect for you. It's up to you to accept those people for their flaws and what they have to offer in your relationship.

Chapter 7

Being disabled may bring your spirits down overtime; it may take you a while to stumble upon someone worth your time. If it's not a person, find a hobby that will awaken a passion within you. Education is also an essential part of your success; it's something worth investing in toward your goals in life.

The people with disabilities in my town mainly work in factories or are cooks and dishwashers, although it all depends on your disability and which kinds of working positions would be best for you.

Learning disabilities can affect our ability to stand for a long time and do specific jobs, focusing on what we should be doing on the job. Being discriminated against happens daily, even though the law states that no one should be refused a job just because of their disability.

To some of us, having a job completes our world; the mere thought of getting up and going to work gives us a sense of purpose and independence. Not depending on anyone for money makes a person feel less disabled; we feel like we can do anything.

I like to think that a disability isn't supposed to hold you back from working and being experienced. You don't see many disabled people in courtrooms or offices. I'm the type of person who would go beyond someone else's beliefs about me to prove them wrong – that I can do it.

I've worked in a day-care, a cookie factory, and I've owned, sold, and rented real estate property. I spent time being a single mother of three, and now, I'm writing this book to prove to you all that my disability doesn't define who I am.

All you need is someone who will lift you during your most challenging times. I had a lot of help from caseworkers, the local department of human services, counselors at my job, at the day-care, overall friends, and people I've run across with great advice.

My husband is my rock, always there for me and supporting me through it all. He is not disabled, but he treats me like we are total equals, which we are, in reality, two humans. Our relationship carries so much love that we always motivate one another.

We planned a lot of trips to keep our life interesting. Adventure sometimes does well, and we are never afraid to live life to the fullest.

Two of our children are disabled, and we always teach them that they can be and do anything. That doesn't stop them from being like the rest; my son is smart as a whip and is better with a computer than I am – he is my genius.

Motivation and dedication are the main things we need. Well, I'd say guidance as well. I don't let my disability stop me from doing anything, and that's what I also teach my kids; if it's a plan and I want to do it, I'm doing it. Nothing will hold me back. With this mindset, I was able to start and accomplish many projects.

All you need in this life is to stick through everything with a little motivation. Plan what you want to achieve, don't let it be simple, and don't need a complicated one. Make it easy to follow but also challenge yourself in the process. How far can you go? Don't force yourself – take things step by step but don't move slowly; life is too short for that.

Thinking about getting into college is important, but make sure you have a guide or a counselor to discuss your disabilities and choose the best path for you. I've attended online colleges and universities. Yes, they are comfortable, but you do have a great responsibility with deadlines and teaching yourself most of the time.

You have to search for what's best for you, either showing up for a class or taking it online. Working online is much more flexible than meeting in a classroom every day. Don't be hung upon a single thing; if it doesn't work for you, try something else. There is something for everyone.

Chapter 8

I f you're in a situation where your kids are disabled, try to be there for them no matter what. Disabled children need your attention more, and giving them an everyday life is the main thing you should be providing.

Your child should grow up in a loving family; that factor is essential for him to be shaped like the right person. If you are motivated, you will do anything in your power to give your children a better life from the one you've experienced.

Your social security check for your disability shouldn't be your only income source; you should develop a plan to keep up with your children's needs. If you don't want to do that, then I suggest you don't have any. Shaping a child into a responsible adult provides them with supplies and makes them appreciate what you do for them. All of the school supplies may leave a big hole in your pocket, but it's worth it; education is a main priority.

Sure, toys aren't necessary, but every child deserves them every once in a while. It brings happiness and joy, which is the main thing we want to see on our children's faces. Love, protect, and support your child, as I stated before but make sure you love yourself and support yourself first. Without that, you're not capable enough to do it for them.

Children are delicate and they mirror their parents; they learn as they grow and how you're raising them is crucial for their development as a young person. Reflect on yourself and the actions you're doing in front of them because they will be repeated; violence is not always the answer. You have to distinguish right from wrong and have talks with them. They will act out less if you have a talk rather than a beating, as per studies.

Everyone needs motivation so take time to engage with them. Your boys may like to play football, basketball and the girls may like to take ballet, dance, or play softball. It's essential to include them in everything, give them a sense of security and support and encourage them. You don't want your child to be antisocial. This could bring them lots of new friends, and with that, they would feel accepted.

Chapter 9

I n this life, you're learning as you go. You never stop learning, and that's the moral of every story; the decisions and actions you make may affect you in the long run. However, staying positive is what you should focus on the most.

Who you are now doesn't mean you will remain in the future; some of us are born into wealthy families, with a silver spoon in our mouths and we always have things handed to us. But you have to realize that if things are handed to you without any hard work, you lose the value of everything; you should experience independence but don't rely on someone else.

God is the one who provides but He can also take away. Everything happens for a reason, and you shouldn't take life for granted. Some of these impressions will be good, and others will be bad. It is all part of the lesson, though.

We are born into an environment in which we need to fight; life is a game. You need to know how to play your cards and play them right; the better your team is, the better the outcome of surrounding yourself with positive people.

A wise woman once told me that people who want to be successful surround themselves with successful people. I find nothing but the truth in that. She also said that people, who want to do nothing, hang around those who do nothing and that fools will hang around fools who always have a negative mindset.

People with a plan drive the world, those who succeed the most believe in themselves, and their ideas reflect how a person should be a fighter. We were placed on this earth with a purpose, and as a human race, we wouldn't have any inventions or innovations without these minds. So, never let anyone tell you that you're not good enough.

Be who you are, don't be ashamed about it, don't accept just right, don't settle but always strive for the best, I believe you can. Test your limits and how far you can go. Rise from the negativity and prosper into positivity.

Chapter 10

Due to my brain deficiency, I've experienced some complications in my growth, such as learning disorders and a speech delay. I'm happy now that I could get a lot better at these things.

I believe that the way other people conduct and behave themselves is mainly influenced by the factors that affected their growth and development early on.

I've learned not to allow any negative energy in my life or my goals. I was a slow learner, but most students thought of my inactiveness as stupidity. I progressed with my education when our class teacher brought up special needs students and our problems more often, which I'm eternally grateful for – that teacher helped me a lot.

Chapter 11

A part of my goal and purpose in life is letting people know about me and my story. You are not alone; when one door closes, another door opens. There are many times when I wanted to give up, but I didn't let it get to me. You must believe in yourself in life. Trust and believe that God is working for you. I am a living testimony.

Chapter 12

When, I had my fourth child, my husband and I were separated. I called my favorite aunt, Leola, who always advised me right. She was always there for me, and her warm words brought me comfort; she would always be there for my other three children and I.

I was on bedrest for my whole pregnancy, and when I told my aunt that I wasn't okay, she told me to rest; she would be there for me. I could vividly remember when my water broke; my husband took me to the hospital.

I had a baby boy. I was excited when I told my mother about my baby. She wanted to move in with my husband and me; although our relationship wasn't the best, my son was my number one priority at the time.

My blood pressure kept going up, and the medications they gave me didn't work at all. The doctor was convinced I would have another seizure. My husband called my family, but sadly, no one came but my aunt, Leola.

I fought with her by my side, and I didn't give up; I could still remember her words, "I love you, don't take her life yet." She was talking to me. "Please, baby, fight it; you have three children and one on the way."

My husband told me that I was a fighter; I came back and had my son. They had to keep me in the hospital for three weeks, and then I was discharged. My children had changed my life. I named my baby son, Oliver Jr, and I felt blessed to have him in my life.

My aunt, Leola, passed away on December 28, 2016. Her passing caused me tremendous pain because I had lost my aunt and best friend. I tried my best to move on, but the bad news kept on going with me, especially also having lost my father-in-law to lung cancer; who died a few weeks after diagnosis. It was the next call I received that struck me again; I had lost my uncle.

My life was a journey full of blessings and hardships, but with God and my own will, I was able to fight through everything and shine the best that I could; with love and respect, I hope you do the same.

Summary

A young girl named Angela Johnson grew up poverty-stricken in Mississippi, suffering from brain damage and debilitating seizures from hyperthyroidism. It's a tough start to life, and many might reasonably ask, what kind of expectations might she have of ever achieving anything? Most children, even her siblings, made fun of her. Adults barely tolerated her.

Then, Angela's story took some unexpected and positive, uplifting – twists and turns that only God Himself could have orchestrated. Her true-life tale is an inspiration to anyone who ever felt that cards were stacked against them. This little girl found the inner strength to beat the odds! Angela grew into adulthood with remarkable perseverance, courage, and unshakable faith in God. It is a powerful testimony that our most precious values come from our souls' dignity, which we see reflected in others, and deep within ourselves.

TO BE CONTINUED!!!!

My Life

Her first autobiography: a memoir by Angela Johnson.

She opens up to the world and shares her testimony of FAITH and COURAGE, as she writes about her life, living with a disability.

Angela Johnson's story is compelling and shows how FAITH, LOVE, AND HOPE conquer ALL.

She shows that DETERMINATION, SACRIFICE and BELIEF IN GOD pay off. All DREAMS can come TRUE.

"GOD has allowed me to share my testimony to help others who live with a disability and mental illness."

Angela Johnson

ABOUT THE AUTHOR

Angela Johnson is a loving wife and mother of four beautiful children.

She works as a licensed Certified Nursing Assistant and Child Development Associate. She resides in Greenwood, MS, with her family.

Made in the USA
Columbia, SC
05 February 2023

11081840R00039